HERBAL SUPPORT FOR HEART HEALTH FOR WOMEN

Discover Holistic Healing: Effective Solutions To   Soothe And Empower For Cardiovascular Well-Being

DR. JEREMY ALLEY

Disclaimer:

The information provided in this book, is intended for general informational purposes only and should not be considered as professional advice.

The author has made every effort to ensure the accuracy of the information presented. However, readers are advised to consult with a qualified healthcare professional before attempting any herbal remedies or making significant changes to their wellness routine. Individual health conditions vary, and what may be suitable for one person may not be appropriate for another.

It is important to note that the author is not in any endorsement deal, partnership, or affiliation with any organization, brand, or company mentioned in this book. Any references to specific products or services are based on the author's personal experience or general knowledge and do not imply an endorsement or promotion of those products or services.

Contents

Overview

A vital component of total well-being is heart health, which is especially important when it comes to women's health. It is crucial to comprehend the particular issues and difficulties that women have about their cardiovascular health as we go more into this subject. With a focus on women specifically, this book attempts to investigate the role of herbal assistance in fostering and sustaining heart health.

Concerning This Book

I feel it is important to give a summary of the content and goals of this book before getting into the details of herbal assistance for women's heart health. The extensive examination of several herbs, their characteristics, and their role in promoting cardiovascular health is what readers may anticipate. There will also be a discussion of useful advice and views on integrating herbal treatments into a comprehensive Heart Health for Women program.

The significance of

Recognizing the significance of heart health is essential to appreciating the role herbal support has in preserving women's cardiovascular health. The particular physiological characteristics that predispose women to particular heart-related disorders will be highlighted in this section. The frequency of heart disease in women and its potential effects on general health and longevity will also be covered.

Function of Herbal Remedies

Herbs have been used for their therapeutic qualities for millennia in many different cultures, and maintaining heart health is only one of those uses. We will look at the particular herbs in this area that are effective in supporting women's cardiovascular health. Readers will learn how herbal medicines can enhance conventional methods for heart health, based on both traditional remedies and contemporary scientific research.

Herbs and Their Beneficial Effects on the Heart

An extensive analysis of particular herbs recognized for their cardiovascular advantages will be covered in this section. Readers will learn about the wide spectrum of plant-based therapies that can improve heart health, from well-known plants like garlic and hawthorn to lesser-known types. We will go over each herb's characteristics, modes of action, and any drawbacks so that readers may make well-informed decisions.

Using Herbs to Help Manage Risk Factors

This section will concentrate on the use of herbal remedies to manage and reduce particular risk factors linked to heart disease in women, in addition to providing general cardiovascular support. The course will cover blood pressure control, cholesterol management, and inflammation management—all essential elements of a holistic approach to heart health.

Using Herbs to Promote a Heart-Healthy Lifestyle

When it comes to health interventions, practicality is essential. Readers will find guidance in this section on incorporating herbal treatments into their daily routines. Knowing how to incorporate herbs into food, teas, and supplements will enable women to actively participate in their heart health journey.

Possible Ideas and Safety Measures

Herbs can provide beneficial support, but it's vital to understand that they might not be right for everyone. We'll talk about some possible pitfalls and safeguards in this section, like drug interactions and personal sensitivities. The knowledge that readers will acquire will help them make well-informed decisions and, where necessary, consult healthcare specialists.

To sum up, this book aims to shed light on the relationship between women's heart health and herbal support. Readers can take the first steps toward holistic heart health by learning about the special requirements of women's cardiovascular systems and investigating the wide variety of herbs available. When people are well-informed, they can make decisions that will improve their health and energy.

CHAPTER ONE

COMPREHENDING THE HEART HEALTH OF WOMEN

Heart health is a vital component of overall well-being, and women have particular considerations that must be taken into account. Although cardiovascular health is typically linked with men, women have unique risks and problems that need to be taken into consideration. Examining the physiological variations, risk factors, and preventative strategies that are essential to preserving heart health is part of understanding women's heart health.

An Overview Of Heart Health

The heart, blood arteries, and blood form the intricate network that makes up the cardiovascular system, which functions to transport nutrients and oxygen throughout the body.

Sustaining cardiovascular health is critical for overall health, and understanding the several aspects that affect heart health is crucial. The foundations of cardiovascular health will be covered in this section, with special emphasis on the value of a healthy heart for both men and women.

Variations In Heart Health By Gender

Men and women have different circulatory systems, but there are noticeable distinctions in the symptoms of heart disease. Different patterns of heart-related problems are influenced by differences in hormones and biology.

Comprehending these gender disparities is essential to customizing efficacious interventions and preventive actions. The subtleties of women's heart health will be examined in this section, along with the elements that set it apart from men's cardiovascular health.

Typical Heart Conditions In Women

Different heart problems can manifest differently in women than in males. For early detection, intervention, and management, it is essential to identify and comprehend these prevalent cardiac diseases. We'll go into great detail about ailments including arrhythmias, heart attacks, heart failure, and coronary artery disease. To promote awareness and preventative care, this section attempts to offer thorough insights into the unique difficulties that women may encounter with heart health.

Herbal Remedies For Heart Health In Women

Growing interest has been seen in using vitamins and herbal therapies to support heart health in recent years. Numerous herbs are thought to have potential advantages for cardiovascular health, and there is growing interest in using them in addition to traditional treatments. The idea of herbal support for women's heart health will be discussed in this section, with a focus on the value of a comprehensive approach to well-being.

Herbs For Heart-Healthy Lifestyle

Traditional medicine has employed a wide variety of herbs to support cardiovascular health. We'll look at some particular herbs in this area that may help women's cardiac health. Hawthorn, garlic, ginger, and turmeric are a few examples. Every plant will be investigated for its supposed benefits, modes of action, and any scientific proof that it contributes to heart health maintenance.

Herbal Remedies For Hormone Regulation

Hormonal changes might affect women's heart health, especially during menopause. Some herbs are thought to support hormonal balance regulation, which may improve cardiovascular health. We shall explore herbal remedies in this section to promote hormonal equilibrium and address the particular difficulties women encounter in this area.

Taking Into Account And Precautions

Herbal medicines have the potential to be beneficial, but you must use caution when using them. The considerations and safety measures for women contemplating herbal support for heart health are outlined in this section.

Topics include possible drug interactions, how much is too much, and why it's best to speak with a doctor before starting a herbal supplement regimen will all be covered.

Including Herbal Support In Daily Activities

Apart from using herbal medicines, women's heart health is greatly influenced by their lifestyle choices.

This section will examine how a holistic lifestyle approach, which includes things like proper food, exercise, stress management, and enough sleep, might incorporate herbal support. Optimizing the advantages of herbal support for heart health can be achieved through a comprehensive strategy.

Women's heart health is a complex topic that necessitates a thorough comprehension of complementary and conventional methods. Herbal support presents opportunities for improving cardiovascular health, but it is important to use these therapies with caution, understanding, and guidance from medical professionals. Through the integration of herbal support and a nutritious lifestyle, women can proactively preserve a robust and resilient heart.

CHAPTER TWO

ESSENTIALS FOR A HEART-HEALTHY LIVES

For general well-being, heart health must be maintained, and for women in particular, a holistic approach is critical. The cornerstones of heart-healthy living include a variety of lifestyle choices that add up to overall cardiovascular health. These include preserving ideal cholesterol levels, controlling blood pressure, and keeping a healthy weight. Support from herbs can be very helpful in strengthening these bases.

Healthy Eating Habits For Cardiovascular Disease

An overall healthy cardiovascular system depends on a well-balanced diet, which is the cornerstone of proper nutrition for heart health. It has been established that several herbs may improve heart health. Garlic, for example, has long been used to lower cholesterol and control blood pressure. Hawthorn berries are also well-known for their cardiovascular advantages, which include enhancing blood flow and fortifying the heart muscle.

It can be advantageous to include a range of heart-healthy herbs in the diet. Curcumin, the main ingredient in turmeric, has anti-inflammatory qualities that may be beneficial to heart health. Because of its well-known antioxidant properties, ginger may help lower oxidative stress in the cardiovascular system. When combined with a healthy diet, these herbs can offer complete support for women's heart health.

The Value Of Frequent Exercise

An essential part of a heart-healthy lifestyle is exercise. Frequent exercise enhances general cardiovascular health, helps control blood pressure, and helps people maintain a healthy weight. Herbal supplements can boost energy levels, lower inflammation, and speed up recovery in addition to exercise regimens. For example, studies have shown that ginseng increases endurance and improves exercise performance, which makes it an excellent supplement for women's fitness programs.

Herbs like ginkgo biloba and hawthorn have the potential to enhance blood circulation, guaranteeing that the heart gets enough oxygen when exercising. It's crucial to remember that speaking with a healthcare provider before adding herbal supplements to a workout regimen is advised to guarantee safety and suitability for certain medical problems.

Techniques For Stress Management

Effective stress management is essential for heart health since prolonged stress is a risk factor for heart disease. Herbal remedies are useful tools for lowering stress. For millennia, people have utilized adaptogenic herbs, such as holy basil and ashwagandha, to assist the body in coping with stress and foster calmness. These herbs may have a beneficial effect on the cardiovascular system by reducing the physiological consequences of stress, which include inflammation and high blood pressure.

Stress management can be further improved by adding relaxation methods like yoga, deep breathing exercises, and meditation to a daily regimen in addition to herbal help. These all-encompassing methods work together to provide a comprehensive plan that supports women's heart health. Including herbal medicines in stress-reduction techniques can offer a holistic and all-natural approach to support cardiovascular health.

an all-encompassing strategy for women's heart health includes addressing the fundamentals of heart-healthy living, combining a balanced diet with herbal support, exercising frequently while taking herbal supplements, and implementing efficient stress-reduction methods with the help of adaptogenic herbs. Through the acceptance of these lifestyle variables and the incorporation of herbal therapies, women can empower themselves to sustain the best possible cardiovascular and general health.

CHAPTER THREE

HERBAL ACUTE HEALTH MEDICATIONS

A vital component of overall health is heart health, and using herbal medicines to promote cardiovascular function is becoming more and more popular. Many civilizations have long used herbal therapy, and many herbs are thought to provide potential heart health advantages. In this investigation, we explore the realm of herbal therapies and consider how they could contribute to cardiovascular wellness.

Herbal Medicine

Phytotherapy, another name for herbal medicine, is the application of plant-based therapies to various health issues. The use of a wide variety of herbs for circulatory support has been a part of traditional treatment systems like Ayurveda and Traditional Chinese Medicine for millennia. Herbs are an interesting source for investigating heart health remedies since they include a wide range of bioactive chemicals that may contribute to their therapeutic effects.

Herbal medication can support a heart-healthy lifestyle, but it should not be used in place of conventional medical care. Several herbs, such as hawthorn, garlic, turmeric, and ginger, are well known for their ability to support cardiovascular function. It is crucial to comprehend these herbs' characteristics and how they affect the cardiovascular system to use them wisely and efficiently.

Selecting The Correct Herbs

The qualities of the herbs and any possible interactions must be carefully considered while choosing the best ones for heart health. For example, hawthorn has long been used to enhance circulation and heart health. It is thought to increase blood vessel dilatation, boost blood flow, and shield the cardiovascular system from free radical damage. Another herb with cardiovascular advantages is garlic, which may also help decrease cholesterol and blood pressure, according to a study.

Curcumin, a substance found in turmeric, a spice with anti-inflammatory qualities, may have cardioprotective effects. Because of its anti-inflammatory and antioxidant qualities, ginger is believed to enhance good blood circulation and lessen inflammation, both of which are linked to heart health. It is best to speak with a healthcare provider before adding herbs to a heart health routine, particularly for people who are taking medication or have pre-existing medical conditions.

Using Herbs In Everyday Living

It can be easy and pleasurable to incorporate herbs into daily living. Herbal teas are a well-liked method of ingesting health-promoting components found in herbs. Making a cup of ginger tea or hawthorn tea, for instance, can be a relaxing daily routine that supports cardiovascular health. Furthermore, adding fresh herbs to food improves flavor and may have health advantages.

Another practical way to include herbal medicines into every day routines is through supplements. Standardized herbal extracts provide a constant and regulated dosage of active ingredients and are offered in liquid or pill form.

However, it's crucial to adhere to dosage recommendations and watch out for any possible drug interactions.

Herbal medicines may be able to help improve the heart health of women.

Although using herbs can be a beneficial supplement to a heart-healthy lifestyle, it's important to use caution and awareness when using them.

Promoting total cardiovascular well-being requires speaking with a healthcare provider and using a holistic strategy that includes regular exercise, a balanced diet, and stress reduction.

CHAPTER FOUR

ESSENTIAL HERBS FOR HEART HEALTH IN WOMEN

Heart health is a fundamental component of overall well-being, and because of particular health considerations, it becomes even more important for women. Herbal support can supplement conventional drug regimens, even though the former is still quite important. Several herbs have shown promise in supporting women's heart health by addressing blood flow, cholesterol, and cardiovascular function in general.

Hawthorn Berry: The Heart Tonic Of Nature

Hawthorn berry is a noteworthy herb for women's heart health because it is a heart tonic inspired by nature. Hawthorn berries have been traditionally used to maintain cardiovascular function. However, due to their ability to increase blood vessel health, regulate blood pressure, and improve overall heart performance, hawthorn berries have gained appeal. Being high in antioxidants, it helps fight oxidative stress, which is frequently connected to cardiac problems. Hawthorn berries may also help blood vessels relax, which would facilitate smoother blood flow and lessen cardiac strain.

Garlic To Support Heart Function

A mainstay of many culinary traditions, garlic is also a major contributor to cardiovascular health. Garlic contains a chemical called allicin, which has been linked to several cardiovascular advantages. It might lessen the risk of atherosclerosis, control cholesterol levels, and lower blood pressure. Adding garlic to food or supplementing with garlic could be a tasty and natural option for women to support heart health. Garlic also improves cardiovascular health in general because of its anti-inflammatory qualities.

Motherwort is a herb that comes up while discussing herbal therapies for women's heart health because of its relaxing effects on the circulatory system.

Motherwort is frequently used to reduce stress and anxiety, and by lowering factors linked to heart strain, it may also indirectly enhance heart health. Motherwort is a useful herb for stress management because of its ability to induce relaxation, which is essential for heart health. Motherwort, especially in the setting of stress-induced heart issues, may help to promote a more resilient and balanced cardiovascular response by soothing the nervous system.

As with any herbal method, women should speak with medical specialists before adding new herbs to their regimen, particularly if they are already on medication or have pre-existing health issues.

Herbal assistance has its uses, but it should be used in addition to conventional medical guidance and care, not as a substitute for it. A balanced diet, regular exercise, stress reduction, and, where appropriate, the judicious addition of herbs with proven cardiovascular benefits are all part of a holistic approach to women's heart health.

Herbal Infusions And Teas

The potential benefits of herbal teas in promoting women's heart health have been acknowledged. These drinks, which come from a variety of plant sources, provide a calm and natural solution for cardiovascular health. Well-known plants like hibiscus, ginger, and hawthorn are frequently used to make heart-healthy infusions.

These herbal teas not only taste delicious and offer solace, but they also support heart health in general.

Making Herbal Tea Blends That Are Heart-Healthy

Making customized herbal tea mixes enables people to customize how they approach heart health. You can increase the tea's overall effectiveness by adding particular herbs that are known to have cardiovascular effects. For example, combining the vasodilatory properties of hawthorn with relaxing herbs like chamomile can result in a blend that promotes stress reduction and heart health. People can find a blend that addresses their specific cardiovascular needs and their taste preferences by experimenting with different herbal combinations.

Combining Herbs To Get The Most Advantages

A key factor in obtaining the most health benefits from herbs is the infusion procedure. Strong herbal elixirs are made by steeping herbs in hot water, which releases water-soluble chemicals. Herbs that help the heart should be infused properly to enhance their effectiveness. Important things to think about are temperature, steeping period, and the proportion of herbs to water. For more difficult herbs, such as hawthorn berries, herbalists frequently suggest a slow boiling technique to ensure that all of the medicinal chemicals are removed.

Tea Recipes To Support Heart Health

Several recipes for herbal tea target women's cardiovascular support in particular. In one such recipe, fragrant herbs like rosemary and mint are combined with hibiscus, a flower recognized for its potential to decrease blood pressure. This blend not only produces a tasty tea but also considers important heart health issues. Moreover, a tea blend with lemon, ginger, and garlic might give you a significant antioxidant boost, which benefits your cardiovascular health in general. Heart-supportive herbs can be a lovely addition to any person's daily routine when used in these recipes.

Herbal teas and infusions that enhance women's heart health provide a comprehensive and pleasurable approach to heart health. Making customized blends and monitoring the infusion procedure guarantee that all of the advantageous ingredients are utilized.

People can experiment and explore a range of herbal choices to find the ideal blend that suits their taste preferences and cardiovascular requirements. Adopting the custom of drinking herbal teas offers proactive measures to support heart health in addition to being a reassuring routine.

CHAPTER FIVE

LIFESTYLE CHANGES FOR HEART REHABILITATION

Adopting a healthy lifestyle can greatly aid in maintaining heart health, which is an essential component of overall well-being. Particularly for women, lifestyle choices are very important in improving cardiovascular health. Preventing heart-related problems requires incorporating heart-healthy habits. We'll look at several lifestyle choices that affect women's heart health in this section.

Heart Health And Restful Sleep

It is impossible to emphasize how important getting enough good sleep is for heart health and general well-being. Heart disease risk is lowered in people who get enough good-quality sleep. Maintaining normal cardiac function is especially crucial for women who prioritize getting quality sleep. The relationship between heart health and sleep will be discussed in this part, with a focus on how important it is to develop appropriate sleep habits.

Strategies For Quitting Smoking

Given that smoking is a known risk factor for heart disease, giving up is essential to enhancing heart health. Similar to men, women who smoke suffer from the cardiovascular effects of their habit, but women-specific techniques can increase the success of quitting. This section will address the effects of smoking on heart health and provide specific recommendations to help women stop smoking and lower their chances of developing heart-related problems.

Sustaining A Healthy Weight

Cardiovascular health depends on maintaining a healthy weight, which is especially important for women. Reaching and maintaining a healthy weight helps reduce the risk of heart disease and its consequences. This section will examine the connection between women's heart health and weight control, shedding light on the need to maintain a balanced diet and level of physical activity for overall health.

Herbal Remedies For Heart Health In Women

Herbal support can play a significant role in a holistic approach to women's heart health, in addition to lifestyle choices.

Since ancient times, herbs have been employed in a variety of conventional therapeutic methods; today, there is growing awareness of the potential advantages of herbs for cardiovascular health.

We'll focus on particular herbs in this area that are well-known for helping to improve women's heart health.

The Advantages Of Taking Herbal Supplements

Due to their possible benefits in promoting heart health, some herbal supplements have become more and more popular. These plants, which include hawthorn, garlic, and turmeric, have qualities that may improve cardiovascular health. Knowing the working principles of these herbal supplements might enable women to choose wisely when adding them to their heart health regimen.

Adaptogenic Plants And The Reduction Of Stress

Heart problems can be exacerbated by prolonged stress, and adaptogenic herbs provide a safe and effective way to reduce stress. Examining the adaptogenic qualities of herbs such as Rhodiola and ashwagandha can provide insight into their possible function in reducing the negative effects of stress on women's heart health.

Herbs High In Antioxidants And Cardiovascular Protection

To shield the cardiovascular system from oxidative stress, antioxidants are essential. Due to their high antioxidant content, herbs like hibiscus and green tea can support heart health in general. This section will look at some herbs' antioxidant qualities and how they could protect women's heart health.

Integration Of Herbal Lifestyle

When incorporating herbal assistance into daily life, each person's unique health demands must be carefully considered.

This section will provide helpful advice on how to smoothly integrate herbal remedies into everyday activities so that women can follow a heart-healthy lifestyle and benefit from these natural therapies.

The complex issue of women's heart health includes lifestyle decisions, sleep patterns, smoking behaviors, and weight control. When used carefully, herbal support can enhance these initiatives and give the cardiovascular system an extra layer of care.

Women can actively engage in behaviors that support a strong and resilient heart by being aware of how these factors interact.

CHAPTER SIX

DISHES FOR A HEART-HEALTHY DIET

For general health, heart health must be maintained at its peak, and adding herbal support to your diet can be a tasty, all-natural method to boost cardiovascular health. With a focus on using herbs recognized for their heart-healthy qualities, this collection of dishes provides a tasty and nourishing way to promote women's heart health.

Smoothies With Herbs To Support The Heart

Heart-healthy herbs can be easily and happily incorporated into your everyday routine with smoothies.

A delightful combination of berries, spinach, and a hint of cayenne pepper to start your day. Berries' antioxidants, spinach's anti-inflammatory qualities, and cayenne's cardiovascular advantages mix to provide a powerful blend that supports heart health. Try experimenting with different herbs to give your smoothie repertoire more depth, such as hawthorn, which is well-known for its beneficial effects on blood circulation.

Heart-Healthy Dressings For Salads

Heart-healthy diets often include salads, and the appropriate dressing can improve the nutritional content and flavor of your greens. Think about combining oregano, garlic, and olive oil to make a vinaigrette. Garlic has anti-inflammatory qualities, oregano provides antioxidants, and olive oil is high in monounsaturated fats. This combo not only makes your salad taste better, but it also strengthens the overall cardiovascular benefits of your diet. Try different herbs, like as basil or rosemary, to provide more flavor and heart-healthy benefits.

Recipes For Main Courses Using Heart-Healthy Herbs

Heart-healthy herbs are a delicious way to put cardiovascular health first in your main course recipes. Marinate lean protein, like chicken or fish, in a mixture of thyme, rosemary, and turmeric to create a flavorful herb-infused roast. Turmeric is well known for its anti-inflammatory qualities, and thyme and rosemary also have antioxidant qualities. This delicious concoction not only entices the palate but also supports heart health by addressing important variables that contribute to cardiovascular health.

As you explore these heart-healthy dishes, keep in mind that maintaining consistency is essential to overall wellness. You can enjoy the tastes of nature and give your heart the support it needs by including these herbal delicacies in your diet.

Including Herbal Support In Day-To-Day Activities

Preserving cardiovascular health is an essential component of general health, and as women age, this becomes increasingly critical. A comprehensive strategy for supporting cardiovascular health may involve incorporating herbal support into daily life. Because of their potential advantages, herbs have been employed in traditional medicine systems for generations. Including herbs in one's regimen can support a heart-healthy lifestyle.

Many herbs have been examined for their possible cardiovascular benefits, including hawthorn, garlic, and turmeric. For example, hawthorn is thought to enhance heart health by encouraging normal blood pressure and blood flow. Garlic has been linked to a reduction in cholesterol levels, while curcumin, the major ingredient in turmeric, has antioxidant and anti-inflammatory qualities that may benefit heart health.

Formulating A Customized Herbal Program

The secret to using herbal support for women's heart health effectively is to customize a regimen to meet each person's needs and preferences. To develop a customized herbal regimen, it is best to speak with a trained herbalist or medical expert. Age, pre-existing medical issues, lifestyle choices, and other factors all influence which herbs and dosages are best for a given person.

Herbs can be incorporated into daily life in several ways, including brewing herbal teas, adding them to meals, or taking supplements. Developing a regimen that fits in with a person's schedule and preferences maximizes the chances of regular use and the possible health advantages of herbal assistance for heart health.

Herbal supplements offer a practical way to add concentrated forms of particular plants into one's lifestyle. However, it's important to pay attention to these supplements' dosage and quality. The supplements are guaranteed to be free of impurities and to contain the appropriate herbal elements thanks to quality assurance and sourcing from reliable suppliers.

Depending on the plant and the person's health, different dosages may apply.

For instance, research indicates that taking garlic extract daily may help control cholesterol.

But for those who want to boost heart health overall, hawthorn supplements might be suggested. A healthcare provider's advice can help determine the right dosage based on personal health objectives and circumstances.

Tracking The Development Of Heart Health

When adding herbal support to one's regimen, it is imperative to regularly assess one's heart health. This entails monitoring vital signs like cholesterol, blood pressure, and general cardiovascular health.

Collaborating with medical professionals enables well-informed decisions to be made on the continuation or modification of herbal supplementation, taking into account the patient's development and any modifications to their health status.

It is crucial to remember that, when necessary, medical assistance cannot be replaced by herbal support.

To make sure that herbal supplements complement their overall treatment plan, women with cardiac conditions—either pre-existing or at risk—should be in constant touch with their healthcare practitioners.

Following the development of heart health gives important information about how effectively herbal assistance works and enables changes to be made as needed to ensure the best possible cardiovascular health.

CHAPTER SEVEN

SUCCESS STORIES AND CASE STUDIES

Experiences from everyday life might offer important insights into how well herbal supplements for women's heart health work. Several case studies demonstrate the benefits of using herbs in comprehensive heart health regimens. These examples show how certain herbs have helped women's cardiovascular outcomes when combined with lifestyle modifications.

Practical Experiences With Herbal Assistance

A more individualized viewpoint is provided by the individual accounts of women who have used herbal treatments in their journey toward heart health. These accounts illuminated the difficulties encountered, the process of making decisions, and the results obtained. Knowing how herbal support works in the real world might encourage people to research these natural options and make wise decisions for their cardiovascular health.

Testimonials From Females Pursuing Heart Health

Women can share their personal experiences of using herbal treatments for heart health through testimonials. These testimonies provide a wide range of experiences, describing the particular herbs used, the advantages said to be obtained, and any difficulties faced.

They urge other women to seek alternate ways to heart health and provide evidence of the possible efficacy of herbal support.

The field of herbal assistance for women's heart health is vibrant and complex. Anecdotal evidence from case studies firsthand accounts, and real-life experiences suggest that herbal medicines can be valuable components of a holistic approach to cardiovascular well-being, even as a scientific study on the effectiveness of different herbs continues. To guarantee individualized and secure interventions, speaking with medical specialists is crucial while making any decisions about one's health.

FINAL VERDICT

herbal assistance contributes significantly to women's heart health.

A comprehensive strategy is required because of the particular difficulties that women encounter, such as daily pressures and hormone variations.

Including herbs such as hawthorn, garlic, ginger, and others can support cardiovascular health in addition to traditional medical treatments.

Conclusion Of Important Ideas

Understanding Women's Heart Health: Menopause, pregnancy, and hormonal changes are some of the factors that affect women's cardiovascular health.

Herbs for Cardiovascular Health: By improving blood vessel health, lowering blood pressure, and lowering cholesterol, hawthorn, garlic, and ginger provide beneficial assistance.

Hormonal Balance and Heart Health: Herbs that address hormonal imbalances, such as black cohosh and dong quai, may have a good effect on heart health.

Mind-Body Connection: Stress Reduction: Among the key factors in preventing heart disease in women is stress management, which is aided by adaptogenic herbs such as holy basil and ashwagandha.

Antioxidant Support for Heart Health: Curcumin, the active ingredient in turmeric, is a powerful antioxidant that supports heart health in general.

Developing Heart-Healthy Lifestyles In Women

A multimodal strategy that incorporates awareness, lifestyle adjustments, and the use of herbal support is needed to empower women to heart-healthy living. Women can be proactive in nurturing their hearts and improving their general well-being by adopting holistic tactics and comprehending the particular characteristics of women's cardiovascular health.